Progesterone: The Superstar of Hormone Balance

Womens Wellness Publishing, LLC
www.womenswellnesspublishing.com
www.facebook.com/wwpublishing

Mention of specific companies or products in this book does not suggest endorsement by the author or publisher. Internet addresses and telephone numbers for resources provided in this book were accurate at the time it went to press.

Cover design by Rebecca Rose

ISBN 978-1-939013-89-7

Note: The information in this book is meant to complement the advice and guidance of your physician, not replace it. It is very important that women who have medical problems be evaluated by a physician. If you are under the care of a physician, you should discuss any major changes in your regimen with him or her. Because this is a book and not a medical consultation, keep in mind that the information presented here may not apply in your particular case. In view of individual medical requirements, new research, and government regulations, it is the responsibility of the reader to validate health practices and treatments with a physician or health service.

Acknowledgements

I want to give a huge thanks to my amazing editors Kendra Chun and Sandra K. Friend for their incredibly helpful assistance with putting this book together. I also greatly appreciate my fantastic Creative Director, Rebecca Richards, as well as Letitia Truslow, my wonderful Director of Media Relations. I enjoyed working with all of them and found their help indispensable in creating this exceptional book for women.

Table of Contents

1

Why Progesterone is Essential to Your Health

Whatever your age and stage of life, maintaining healthy progesterone levels is crucial to your female health and overall well-being. Deficiency of this vital hormone can produce uncomfortable and even dangerous symptoms, and contribute to many female health issues at all stages of life. Progesterone even affects our emotional balance and our ability to handle the stresses that we encounter in our day-to-day living. As a physician, I have seen firsthand how beneficial having an optimal level of this important hormone is for the female body. I've developed programs for my patients that have successfully helped to support their own production of progesterone as well worked with bioidentical progesterone therapy. I will be sharing much of this information with you in this book.

Let's start by discussing some important facts about progesterone.

What is Progesterone

Progesterone is one of the two major female sex hormones. Along with estrogen, it is responsible for many of the traits that we consider to be uniquely female. Progesterone is the yang to estrogen's yin. While estrogen is a growth-stimulating and expansive hormone, progesterone tends to limit the growth of tissue, therefore having a more contractive or yangizing effect on the body.

Often a "silent partner," progesterone is produced in the ovaries in women, with some production in the adrenals. It is produced in the ovaries in women, and both men and women produce some progesterone in the adrenals. During pregnancy, as the fetus matures, the placenta produces large amounts of progesterone (the name actually means "for gestation").

Men produce a small but significant amount throughout life, comparable to how much a woman makes after age forty-five or fifty. In men, the main function of progesterone seems to be helping to maintain libido.

In women, progesterone acts together with estrogen to facilitate menstruation and pregnancy. A healthy balance of these two hormones is also important for health and mood in women. Sufficient progesterone is necessary to support the ability to remain calm under pressure, the ability to concentrate, physical energy, as well as a balanced emotional state. Aging, too rigorous exercise, stress, and poor health cause the production of progesterone to diminish, affecting health as well as performance.

Health conditions affected by a lack of adequate progesterone include elevated levels of estrogen (estrogen dominance), hot flashes, endometrial cancer, heart disease, and osteoporosis. Supplementation with progesterone, whether natural or synthetic, helps to prevent and correct these conditions.

I first started to use bioidentical progesterone as well as a nutritional program to help support a woman's own production of progesterone with my PMS and premenopause patients. The results were so positive, and often occurred so rapidly, usually within one or two menstrual cycles, that I began to expand the program to many of the women I worked with including many postmenopausal women. Over the years, my program has helped thousands of female patients, often with great and, even, dramatic results.

I wrote this book to share my program with you so that you, too, can experience the incredible benefits that having optimal levels of progesterone provides for our bodies. I have compiled a helpful list of progesterone's peak-performance and health benefits for women to provide you with a summary of the how supportive progesterone is for women's health and wellness.

Benefits of Progesterone for Women

Peak-Performance Benefits
- Increased physical vitality and stamina (improves sleep patterns)
- Enhanced mental clarity and acuity
- Increased ability to get along with other people (balances mood)
- Increased ability to remain calm under pressure

Health Benefits of Progesterone
- Helps control excessive and irregular menstrual bleeding during perimenopause
- Helps prevent health problems related to high estrogen levels, such as endometrial hyperplasia and uterine fibroids
- Reduces hot flashes
- Helps prevent uterine cancer
- Helps prevent osteoporosis
- Increases libido
- Aids in the healing of certain types of nerve disease
- Improves sleep patterns
- Reduces Brain Fog

2

Understanding the Role of Progesterone in the Body

Progesterone, along with estrogen, is one of your primary female hormones. These hormones are derived directly from pregnenolone, the "mother" hormone from which all the other sex hormones are produced. The chemical structure of progesterone is also similar to that of the other sex hormones, such as estrogen and testosterone.

Progesterone is primarily produced by the corpus luteum of the ovary. This is the "yellow body" that is created during the second half of your menstrual cycle. If pregnancy occurs, progesterone is also secreted by the placenta.

While estrogen causes tissues to grow and thicken, progesterone has more of a maturing and limiting effect on tissues. For example, progesterone prevents the uterine lining from becoming too thick during the second half of the menstrual cycle and even, over time, from becoming cancerous. Progesterone also prevents menstrual bleeding from becoming too profuse or long lasting.

It also stimulates secretions throughout your body. For example, when progesterone production is stimulated during the second half of your menstrual cycle, the lining of your uterus secretes nutrients critical to the development of an embryo. Similarly, progesterone also causes secretion of those cells in your breasts that are necessary to produce breast milk.

Progesterone has a balancing effect on estrogen in many other ways, affecting many physical and chemical functions in the body. For example, progesterone acts as a sedative to the nervous system. Its effect is calming and sedating. In contrast, estrogen has a stimulatory effect on the nervous system. In fact, increased levels of estrogen can trigger anxiety, irritability, and mood swings.

Estrogen lowers blood sugar levels while progesterone increases them. Additionally, estrogen tends to cause salt and fluid retention, while progesterone acts as a natural diuretic. For example, estrogen increases body fat while progesterone helps you burn fat for energy. This is why it is so critical to ensure that all of your hormone levels are in proper balance.

Progesterone plays a key role in menstruation and pregnancy. The purpose of the menstrual cycle is to prepare the female body for conception and possible pregnancy. The entire process of menstruation depends on the balanced interaction of several hormones, especially estrogen and progesterone. Working together, they prepare the lining of the uterus (the endometrium) to receive a fertilized egg, should pregnancy occur. The surge of progesterone after an egg is released from the ovarian follicle greatly stimulates the libido, which increases the likelihood that a sperm will enter the female and unite with the egg.

The increase in production of progesterone at mid-cycle causes a rise in body temperature of about 0.5° to 1°F, which many women monitor to identify when ovulation is most likely to occur and, therefore, the days when they are fertile. If the egg does not unite with a sperm, progesterone output declines. This stimulates the cells of the uterine lining to slough off and be excreted, which is experienced as menstruation. A rapid decline in progesterone triggers your monthly menstrual bleeding.

During your monthly cycle, the level of progesterone rises and falls dramatically, from 2-3 mg per day in the first half of the month, to 22 mg per day in the second half of the month. For some women, this number can be as high as 30 mg per day.

Should pregnancy occur, the placenta also begins to produce progesterone, greatly adding to the amount of hormone in circulation. By the fourth month of gestation, a woman produces 10 times her normal amount. During the last months of pregnancy, daily production can be as high as 300-400 mg a day. To appreciate the significance of this quantity, consider that the various hormones produced within the body are usually measured in micrograms (a thousand-fold less).

Besides its role in the menstrual cycle, progesterone participates in several other vital functions. These other metabolic actions are especially important because they help women to maintain general good health and help prevent disease. For instance, progesterone helps keep blood sugar levels normal, aids the activity of the thyroid, and functions as a natural diuretic. It also normalizes zinc and copper levels, promotes the metabolic conversion of fat into energy, and normalizes blood clotting.

Having sufficient levels of progesterone also helps to prevent the development of a variety of diseases. For example, progesterone prevents the uterine lining from becoming too thick during the second half of the menstrual cycle and even, over time, from becoming cancerous. Progesterone also prevents menstrual bleeding from becoming too profuse or long lasting.

3

Hormone Balance Through the Years

As mentioned in the last chapter, when estrogen and progesterone are produced in normal amounts, they have opposing and complementary effects on your body. However, when these hormones are out of balance, your body and your health can pay a dear price.

For now, what you need to know is that proper balance between estrogen and progesterone is the key to a balanced mood, healthy sex drive, ideal body weight, and soft, firm skin. They can also offer protection against heart disease, stroke, osteoporosis, and even Alzheimer's disease.

Estrogen and progesterone produce these positive effects in your body by binding to hormone receptors in tissues in your uterus, breasts, blood vessels, brain, bones and heart, as well as many other tissues. When a hormone reaches its target tissue, it binds to these receptor cells like a key fitting into a lock. When binding occurs, the hormone transmits its chemical message, causing a change in the tissue. In fact, the health of all of the tissues in your body is very sensitive to the healthy balance between estrogen and progesterone. Nowhere is this balance more evident or more critical than your menstrual cycle.

For example, hormones are at their peak during your younger years, when you are menstruating regularly. However, as you reach your 40's, your hormones often go haywire, either producing too much or too little estrogen while the production of progesterone begins to decline. This is a key sign that you are entering the menopause transition. Eventually, every woman ends up with diminished hormone levels, signaling the end of her periods and the start of menopause.

To better understand this natural transition of our production of progesterone from menstruation to menopause. Let's take a look at each stage individually.

The Normal Menstrual Cycle

To fully understand a normal menstrual cycle, you should first know why menstruation even occurs. Menstruation refers to the monthly shedding of the uterine lining. Every month, as your uterus prepares a home for a new baby, it creates a thick, blood-rich lining in which to cushion the fertilized egg.

If conception occurs, the egg will implant itself in this cushion within a week or so. If pregnancy does not occur, the cushion is no longer necessary, and your uterus cleanses itself of the unnecessary lining, making room for a new cushion to be created the next month. This monthly build up and break down of the uterine lining is controlled by hormones.

To trigger the start of your menstrual cycle, your hypothalamus and pituitary glands secrete a hormone (called FSH) that stimulates the follicle surrounding each egg in your ovaries and causes an egg to mature. During this process, the follicle produces increasingly high levels of estrogen. Your ovaries then produce estradiol, while your adrenal glands, triangular shaped organs resting atop each kidney, produce the weaker estrone form of estrogen.

At mid-cycle, a second hormone called the luteinizing hormone (LH) is produced by the pituitary gland. LH triggers the expulsion of the egg from the ovarian follicle. It also increases the synthesis of prostaglandins, short-lived hormones that are needed for this process to occur. Once ovulation has occurred, the egg leaves the ovary and travels down the fallopian tube to the uterus, where pregnancy can occur.

Both estrogen and progesterone are produced during this second half of the cycle by the corpus luteum. This is the structure that develops from the ruptured ovarian follicle after the egg is released from the ovary. The production of progesterone actually predominates during the second half of the cycle.

If the egg is not fertilized, both progesterone and estrogen production decline rapidly, triggering menstruation. It can take three to five days for your body to completely shed the uterine lining. Once it is complete, the hormone cycle starts all over again, with estrogen being produced during the entire menstrual cycle, and progesterone only produced during the second half of the cycle.

The Menopause Transition

Unfortunately, the balance between estrogen and progesterone does not remain intact as a woman ages. By the time you are in your 30's, progesterone production begins to decline. Having an irregular menstrual cycle can also affect your progesterone production. As you enter your 40's, you may notice that the symptoms preceding your periods, as well as the length of the menstrual cycle and the amount of blood lost, will begin to change. This often signals the beginning of the menopause transition.

There are several variables associated with the menopause transition. It can occur as early as the mid-30's or as late as the upper 50's. Plus, it can last anywhere from one year to as long as five or six years. But what remains consistent is the wild hormonal fluctuations that occur. These fluctuations are the hallmark of the menopause transition.

Phase One: Premenopause

The first phase of the transition is premenopause. This phase is often marked by PMS symptoms such as irritability, anxiety, and bloating, as well as weight gain, fibroid tumors, endometriosis, breast tenderness, difficulty conceiving, and even mental fog and concentration problems.

During this time, your estrogen levels can fluctuate. For some women, their levels are too high, while other women will have normal to even lower levels of estrogen production. You also ovulate less frequently, which means that you are also producing less progesterone. Often, the progesterone levels are relatively deficient and unbalanced in relationship to the estrogen levels.

During this same time, your ovaries are beginning to age, actually undergoing physical and structural changes. They begin to shrink and become less responsive to the hypothalamic-pituitary signals. Additionally, you have much fewer eggs available to mature, and the eggs you do have left are older and less functional. This situation often prevents a follicle from maturing enough to expel an egg. When this happens, the second half of the menstrual cycle never kicks in properly, so progesterone isn't adequately produced. As a result, you often are left with too much estrogen and not enough progesterone – or estrogen dominance.

Estrogen dominance is often the cause of symptoms women experience during the pre-menopause phase of the transition. Estrogen dominance is marked by periods of heavy and/ or irregular bleeding when the uterus sloughs off a lining that has been thickened by too much estrogen. This can occur either as a pattern of heavy, prolonged menstrual bleeding or irregular bleeding and spotting. Some women also have mid-cycle bleeding and pain during this time, depending on their underlying gynecological issues.

Some women also develop fibroid tumors during this time. Fibroid tumors are benign growths that usually form on the uterine wall. They can grow so large that in addition to causing heavy or irregular bleeding, they may also put pressure on the bladder or intestines, causing discomfort, frequent urination, or changes in bowel routines in some women. In some cases, they can become so large that a woman can appear to be in her second trimester of pregnancy! Other problems during premenopause include worsening of endometriosis related pain, as well as the appearance of ovarian and breast cysts, tenderness, fluid retention, and bloating – all due to the shift towards estrogen dominance.

Eventually, this irregular and/or heavy bleeding will begin to taper off, signaling the start of phase two of the menopause transition—perimenopause.

Phase Two: Perimenopause

This decline continues in perimenopause, when changes occur in both the length of the menstrual cycle and the amount of blood lost. Often, this occurs during your mid-to-late 40's, although the age can vary greatly.

Some women may skip phase one altogether and only experience perimenopause. Like premenopause, perimenopause can also be marked by wildly fluctuating hormones, weight gain and irregular periods. Because estrogen levels are starting to decline significantly during this phase, you may also start to experience some menopause symptoms, such as hot flashes, insomnia, night sweats, decreased libido, and fatigue, even if you are still having menstrual periods.

However, unlike premenopause, your production of estrogen and testosterone are definitely diminishing. This can occur over several years. Additionally, you have less and less frequent ovulation, which means lower and lower levels of progesterone. This creates a state of hormone deficiency (especially estrogen), rather than a relative excess of estrogen as compared to progesterone, as seen with estrogen dominance.

Progesterone levels are often greatly diminished by perimenopause.

Instead of the heavy menstrual bleeding that occurs during premenopause, perimenopause is marked by fewer and fewer periods. Often, they will be spaced further and further apart, with less bleeding during each occurrence. Eventually, menstruation ceases entirely as you complete your transition into menopause.

Menopause: The Change of Life

Some lucky women—about 10 percent—make this transition easily. They simply have fewer and fewer periods, mild to no symptoms, a couple of hot flashes and their periods stop. However, you aren't officially in menopause until you have not had a period for at least one year. For 95 percent of women, this takes place between the ages of 45 and 55, with most women reaching menopause right around age 50 or 51.

When a woman enters menopause, her levels of estrogen, progesterone, and testosterone decline to levels that no longer support menstruation. While women after menopause can occasionally experience a bleeding episode, essentially menstruation ceases. In addition, other more wide-ranging shifts occur in her physical, chemical, and energetic makeup.

The patients I've seen in my practice who have the easiest transition into menopause are those who are already on a strong preventive nutritional program. But frankly, most doctors don't usually see this healthy transition. Unless a woman is one of the lucky 10 percent or is on a strong preventive nutritional program, she is more likely to begin experiencing health problems due to estrogen-progesterone imbalances.

By the time menstrual periods stop, estrogen production has diminished by as much as 75 to 90 percent, progesterone production has virtually ceased, and the production of androgens—male hormones that stimulate sex drive—are up to 50 percent lower. Simply put, menopause is a state of hormone deficiency.

This life change is due to normal aging of ovaries and egg follicles. In the menopause transition and the early stages of menopause, the ovarian follicles begin to atrophy, reducing your ability to produce estrogen. You ovulate less frequently, thereby producing less progesterone or no progesterone at all during certain months. In an attempt to force the ovaries to manufacture more hormones, the levels of the pituitary hormone FSH (follicle-stimulating hormone) become elevated. FSH is the hormone that triggers follicular function in the ovaries.

Paradoxically, your ovaries may go into overdrive in response to the pituitary stimulation. In fact, for a time, your ovaries may produce high levels of estrogen until they are finally exhausted. When this occurs, estrogen levels may drop permanently, and menstruation ceases. As a result, hormonal levels may fluctuate during this time, and the balance between estrogen and progesterone is disrupted.

Previously, the medical textbooks indicated that a woman was born with a set number of eggs and that over time, as the ovaries aged and shrank and there were fewer eggs that could be utilized, a woman would eventually just naturally slip into menopause. But new research from the journal *Nature* has shown just how wrong this is.

Researchers at Massachusetts General Hospital in Boston have discovered special stem cells that, until now, have been overlooked, allow women to continue to produce eggs throughout their life. The eggs derived from these cells also form new follicles (where the eggs ripen and mature). It is these follicles within the ovary that, together with the adrenal glands, are responsible for hormone production. This may be a partial explanation for why the exciting approach that I am sharing with you in this book can offer so much potential to better optimize your hormone production and balance, no matter what your age, and allow you to enjoy a much more vital and healthy life.

During menopause, the ovaries and adrenal glands continue to produce estrone (a lower potency estrogen) and the liver produces some estriol (another weak form of estrogen). And while their action is not nearly as strong as the hormones produced before menopause, these hormones do continue to provide some support for the bones, breasts, brain, heart, and vaginal tissues.

The problems that often accompany menopause — hot flashes, insomnia, vaginal dryness, painful intercourse, loss of libido, vaginal and bladder infections, loss of muscle and skin tone, achy joints, brittle bones, fatigue, and mental confusion--are unpleasant, distressing, and can prevent us from living life to the fullest. Some naturally disappear in a few years; others do not. The good news is that with my program you don't have to accept these as a "natural" part of the life cycle.

How Lifestyle and Health Affect Progesterone Levels

Progesterone production diminishes with age, but its output is also influenced by lifestyle factors as well. Digestive capability and liver function will also influence progesterone levels. Following is a discussion of how all these factors affect progesterone production.

Exercise

Women who exercise a great deal and consequently have low levels of body fat may eventually no longer ovulate once a month. This is most frequently seen in female athletes, dancers, and other extremely physically active women. When this happens, the body does not have sufficient levels of cholesterol to manufacture the hormones needed to cause ovulation to occur. And when a women is anovulatory, the ovaries cease making progesterone.

Stress

Physical, emotional, and mental stress can inhibit the production of progesterone. When the body is put through long-term physical stress, as is true of athletes, the daily rhythms of hormone production, including progesterone, can be disrupted.

Physiological Factors

People with poor digestion are unable to absorb certain hormone precursors, which limits hormone production. Poor liver function, with reduced activity of liver enzyme systems, can also lead to lower levels of progesterone, as the conversion of pregnenolone to DHEA and progesterone is impaired.

Summary

Hormones, primarily secreted by the glands, or endocrine system, are the chemical messengers of the body. They perform myriad functions and are divided into several categories. The series of chemical reactions that produce the sex hormones begins with cholesterol. The three major sex hormones are estrogen, progesterone, and testosterone. The two precursor hormones, from which these and all other sex hormones are made, are pregnenolone and DHEA. An adequate, balanced supply of all five sex hormones is necessary for optimal health.

Defining where you are in the four distinct phases of a woman's life—menstruation, premenopause, peri-menopause, or menopause—will help you better understand your own hormonal makeup, and help you decide which hormones you need to focus on to achieve great health and well-being.

In the next few chapters, I'll share with you how our progesterone levels affect all aspects of our physical and emotional health and well-being.

4

Progesterone and Peak Performance

As one of the major female sex hormones, progesterone affects many body systems and tissues. Yet, It also greatly affects your mood, emotions, and mental clarity. In fact, having optimal levels of progesterone are very important to be able to enjoy a high quality of life. In this chapter, I discuss many of these traits that optimal levels of progesterone support.

Physical Vitality and Stamina

Progesterone therapy during perimenopause and the postmenopausal years can potentially reduce fatigue and increase energy by improving sleep quality. An often-noted side effect of progesterone therapy is that it causes sleepiness. In fact, this hormone is thought to restore normal sleep patterns. Various reasons for this have been suggested, related to its ability to calm and act as a tranquilizer.

Mental Clarity and Acuity

Mental acuity and the ability to concentrate depend on adequate levels of progesterone within the body. After menopause has occured, when ovarian progesterone production has ceased, maintaining youthful amounts can be crucial for continuing to meet job requirements. A person working as a lawyer or an accountant for forty years needs to think as quickly and accurately at the end of his or her career as when it began.

Progesterone treatment has been shown to increase mental ability. A study published in the *British Medical Journal* followed twenty-three women for four months. Each woman received 300 mg of oral progesterone daily for two continuous months. Those women receiving treatment had a clear improvement in concentration.

Similar increases in mental acuity and the ability to remain focused on a subject have also been found in premenopausal and postmenopausal women. Progesterone has also been effective in elderly people who have become senile, helping them to regain some degree of mental alertness.

This effect of progesterone may be due to several factors involving brain function. Relatively large amounts of progesterone are present in brain cells, twenty times greater than in the blood. It is thought that progesterone enhances the amount of oxygen in the cells of the brain, thereby increasing mental acuity.

The Ability to Get Along With Other People

Progesterone has a significant effect on mood, thereby affecting how women relate to others both at home and in work situations. For example, pregnant women, who produce great quantities of progesterone, tend to have an exceptional sense of well-being. Conversely, after birth, when progesterone production suddenly plummets, some women may develop postpartum depression.

Low progesterone levels also contribute to the emotional symptoms associated with PMS, including anxiety, irritability, and depression. Treatment with progesterone has been found to relieve these symptoms. In a study published in the *Journal of Assisted Reproduction and Genetics*, twenty-five women with severe PMS and seventeen reproductive-age females participated in a controlled trial. Treatment consisted of a 200 mg vaginal progesterone suppository, taken twice daily. The researchers observed that the women receiving the progesterone reported significant improvement in nervous symptoms.

The association of progesterone with mood swings is evident when considering the years in a woman's life in which they most commonly occur. About 60 percent of women have mild to moderate PMS in their late thirties and forties. These are the pre and perimenopausal years, when hormone production becomes irregular. An additional 15 to 20 percent of women will have symptoms severe enough to disrupt functioning both at home and at work.

However, with the onset of menopause, when the ovarian production of progesterone and estrogen, greatly diminishes, these symptoms permanently subside. Furthermore, cross-cultural epidemiological studies worldwide show that anxiety disorders and depression are two to three times more common in women than they are in men.

One way in which progesterone may influence mood is through its direct effect on neurotransmitters. According to an article appearing in the *International Journal of Fertility*, changes in levels of progesterone have been shown to influence the production and breakdown of brain chemicals that modulate mood. These include the central nervous system neurotransmitters dopamine, serotonin, norepinephrine, and acetylcholine.

Both the peripheral and the central nervous systems have hormone receptors and react to changes in the level of progesterone. It is thought that the ability of progesterone to generate a sense of well-being depends on this brain-related activity.

Any woman considering taking progesterone for its performance as well as health benefits should consider using natural progesterone rather than the progestins. In my own clinical practice, I have found it to be better tolerated and cause less detrimental effects on such important performance traits as physical energy and mood than the synthetic forms. Research studies are beginning to confirm its benefits. Be sure to consult with a physician who is knowledgeable about how to use natural progesterone.

The Ability to Remain Calm Under Pressure

Being able to remain calm under stress is a capability rarely listed on a resume but a prerequisite for many jobs nonetheless. Progesterone helps promote this natural calm. It is sometimes referred to as a natural tranquilizer, as it has a calming and even mildly sedating effect. Taken in high dosages, it has been used as an anesthetic.

It is thought that this calming effect is due to the conversion of progesterone into substances that slow activity at GABA receptors. GABA (gamma amino-butyric acid) is an amino acid that inhibits neuro transmitters (chemicals that relay information from one part of the brain to another) and has a calming effect. While progesterone has a sedating effect on its own, having a balance between estrogen and progesterone levels is crucial for remaining even-tempered under pressure.

5

Progesterone Deficiency During Premenopause

During the premenopause, the transitional years preceding menopause, a woman will sometimes produce elevated levels of estrogen as compared with progesterone, which is more likely to be produced in normal or low amounts. Women during this time also have fewer ovulatory menstrual cycles.

If you are in premenopause, there are a wide variety of negative health issues that can often result from decreased levels of progesterone These include mood swings, irritability, headaches, fluid retention in the tissues, irregular or heavy menstrual bleeding, and swelling of the breasts premenstrually. Progesterone therapy can help keep these conditions in check.

Elevated levels of estrogen can also overstimulate the growth of the uterine lining and the outer muscular tissue of the uterus, causing the growth of benign tumors called fibroids. Both of these conditions can cause heavy menstrual bleeding, which can, if untreated, lead to severe anemia. Other estrogen dominant related conditions include endometriosis and ovarian cysts.

Elevated estrogen levels can also stimulate a potentially precancerous condition called endometrial hyperplasia. According to a study published in *Fertility and Sterility*, low doses of progesterone are able to control this growth. The study group was comprised of 157 symptomatic postmenopausal women, who were given from 1.5 to 3 mg of estrogen along with 200 to 300 mg of progesterone. Treatment was monitored for a minimum of five years. Cell division was consistently reduced after nine or more days of progesterone use. Elevated levels of estrogen also stimulate the growth of endometrial (uterine) cancer.

Let's take a more in-depth look at the issues affecting decreased levels of progesterone during this time of transition.

Progesterone Imbalances

As one of the major female sex hormones, progesterone affects many body systems and tissues. Decreased levels of this crucial hormone can trigger a wide variety of negative health conditions, ranging from the discomfort of PMS to more life-threatening conditions, such as uterine cancer.

PMS

Premenstrual syndrome (PMS) is thought to be a result of hormonal changes, diet, and lifestyle. Studies have shown that women with PMS tend to have relatively high levels of estrogen and relatively low levels of progesterone.

Low progesterone levels play a particularly large role in the emotional symptoms associated with PMS, including anxiety, irritability, and depression. In fact, progesterone has a significant effect on mood. For example, pregnant women, who produce abundant quantities of progesterone, tend to have an exceptional sense of well-being. Unfortunately, after childbirth, when progesterone production greatly plummets, some women may develop postpartum depression.

The association of progesterone with mood swings is evident when considering the years in a woman's life in which they most commonly occur. About 60 percent of women have mild to moderate PMS in their late 30's and 40's. For many women, this is a time when their hormone production begins to go out of balance. An additional 15-20 percent of women will have symptoms severe enough to disrupt their ability to function both at home and at work.

Fortunately, increasing progesterone through proper diet, exercise, and the right combination of nutrients (and in severe cases, the use of natural progesterone) can ease most, if not all, PMS-related symptoms.

Ovarian Cysts

During normal ovulation, a follicle (the fluid-filled structure that houses an egg before it's released into the fallopian tube) grows to a certain size and then ruptures, releasing the egg. The follicle is then converted into a larger structure, the corpus luteum, which produces both estrogen and progesterone, needed to promote proper growth and maturation of your uterine lining during the second half of your menstrual cycle.

An ovarian cyst forms when the follicle continues to grow, instead of releasing the egg and dissolving like it's supposed to. In other words, the cyst is a failed ovulation, and as such, is a clear indicator that you aren't producing the proper levels of progesterone.

Ovarian cysts are so common that conventional medicine considers them normal. In fact, most cysts do go away on their own within a couple of months. In the event they don't go away, your treatment options aren't so positive—surgically draining, cauterizing, or removing the cyst (along with a section of the ovary); removing the ovary; and/or taking synthetic hormones—all of which only treat the symptoms, not the cause.

Fortunately, increasing your progesterone levels will likely help to reduce or even eliminate symptoms and help cause the cysts to shrink.

Benign Breast Disease

Benign breast disease is a catch-all term for changes in the breast that aren't cancer. According to the American Cancer Society, nine out of 10 women have some type of benign breast disease at some point in their lives. Often, it manifests as breast swelling, pain, and engorgement that can last several days to two weeks during each cycle. In many cases, women complain that their breasts are so tender they can't bear to have them touched. Some women even have to stop running during this period because of the pain.

One of my patients, Jane, was a 38-year-old woman who suffered from cystic changes in her breast, as well as breast swelling and pain for one week prior to the start of her menstrual periods. Her breast swelling and engorgement were so pronounced that she had to buy a larger bra just for this time of the month.

She loved to jog and would run four miles each day as her preferred exercise, except during the time just before her period, when her breast tenderness made running too difficult. She also noticed abdominal bloating, some swelling in her fingers (which made it more difficult for her to take her rings on and off her fingers), and a tendency toward mood swings and crankiness with her husband. Luckily, her symptoms subsided dramatically with the use of my diet and nutritional recommendations.

Hyperplasia and Endometrial (Uterine) Cancer

Endometrial hyperplasia usually affects women between the ages of 50 and 70. In some women, this can be a pre-cancerous condition, in which there is an overgrowth of the cells of the uterine lining, or endometrium (a precursor to endometrial or uterine cancer). In the early stages, there may not be any symptoms, but as the condition progresses, more common symptoms like abnormal vaginal bleeding may occur.

Prevention of endometrial cancer is the primary reason physicians prescribe progesterone. This became evident several decades ago when the incidence of uterine cancer increased in American women who were prescribed unopposed estrogen. Estrogen use fell into decline among the menopausal female population until studies showed that combined estrogen therapy could protect women from the development of this cancer. Without the addition of progesterone to an estrogen treatment regimen, the incidence of endometrial (uterine) cancer increases four- to eight-fold in women with an intact uterus.

I first saw Amanda when she was 40 years old. At that time, she was suffering from mood swings, irritability, bloating, and sugar cravings due to the PMS that had occurred after the birth of her second child. Her PMS symptoms resolved relatively quickly on my nutritional and supplement program and she was able to handle her day-to-day routine without suffering from PMS.

At age 48, Amanda consulted me again. She explained that she had felt extremely well and her menstrual cycles had been normal until the past year when she began to transition into a new phase of her life—premenopause. At that time, her menstrual periods, which had been regular (4-5 days in length, with a moderate amount of bleeding) had now become much heavier, lasted longer, and were more irregular.

She sought help from her gynecologist, who did an endometrial biopsy and told her that she had endometrial hyperplasia, which needed to be watched carefully and treated so that it did not progress to endometrial cancer. He also told her that the condition was caused by her estrogen levels being too high without sufficient production of progesterone.

Amanda asked me if she could resolve this problem using natural healing methods, as she had done with her PMS. I explained to her that with the use of diet and a nutritional supplement program—including natural, biochemically identical progesterone—we could absolutely bring her hormones back into a healthy balance.

Some six months later, I received a very excited phone call from Susan, telling me that upon retesting, her endometrial hyperplasia had totally resolved, and her uterine lining was now normal.

In summary, progesterone therapy can definitely be of great benefit during the premenopause when women are no longer producing the same amount of progesterone that they did during their active reproductive years. Progesterone therapy can help to protect a woman during this sensitive time from the many health conditions that can arise from estrogen dominance.

6

Progesterone Deficiency During Perimenopause and Menopause

During the perimenopause and menopause years, the side effects of decreased progesterone levels continue to plague many women. Not only does progesterone deficiency intensify the symptoms of menopause, but it is also a risk factor for heart disease, osteoporosis, and even certain nerve diseases. In this chapter, I discuss these symptoms as well as fascinating research on how progesterone therapy helps to relieve these debilitating symptoms.

Hot Flashes

Between 15-20 percent of women who are making the transition into menopause experience hot flashes, even while they're still having fairly regular menstrual periods. They may also experience heavy bleeding and premenstrual tension.

Unfortunately, estrogen replacement therapy (ERT) cannot be used to suppress hot flashes because many of these women have times when they produce higher than normal levels of estrogen and often are not ovulating regularly. Thus, ERT used alone could actually intensify the preexisting state of hormonal imbalance.

Happily, progesterone used alone can relieve hot flashes and other vasomotor symptoms in about 60-80 percent of women. Because of its sedative and calming effects, progesterone is also useful in treating menopausal mood swings.

Unfortunately, progesterone is not particularly useful for the treatment of vaginal atrophy or vaginal and bladder infections due to thinning of the mucous membranes since these symptoms are related to estrogen deficiency.

Insomnia

Women deficient in progesterone often have trouble falling or staying asleep. Fortunately, increasing your levels of this hormone can help to restore normal sleep patterns. In fact, progesterone therapy during perimenopause and the postmenopausal years can potentially reduce fatigue and increase energy by improving sleep quality.

Another reason for progesterone's sleep benefits is that it helps to boost and support the effects of GABA (gamma-aminobutyric acid), a calming, inhibitory neurotransmitter, a chemical that relays information from one part of your brain to another. Some women can even benefit by using GABA supplementation during the menopause.

Decreased Sex Drive

Progesterone levels are an important component of your ability to maintain your libido, or sex drive. This is thought to occur through progesterone's effect on the brain, as libido is primarily a brain function. This was observed in one study by John Lee, M.D., that was primarily designed to assess the benefit of progesterone on bone health. In conducting a study of 100 postmenopausal women for three years, Dr. Lee found that one of the effects of treatment was a restoration of libido to normal levels.

This is thought to occur through progesterone's effect on the brain, as libido is primarily a brain function. Animal studies have demonstrated that while estrogen readies the brain cells involved with libido, progesterone is the hormone that activates them.

Certainly for most women, having fulfilling sexual activity is an essential part of life. Progesterone offers one way to restore this ability in those women who have experienced a decline in this function

Brain Fog

Mental acuity and the ability to concentrate depend on adequate progesterone levels within the body. After menopause, when ovarian progesterone production has ceased, many women experience brain fog, periods of forgetfulness, and difficulty remembering names, phone numbers, etc.

Progesterone has also been effective in elderly people who have become senile, helping them to regain some degree of mental alertness. This effect of progesterone may be due to several factors involving brain function. Relatively large amounts of progesterone are present in brain cells, 20 times greater than in the blood. It is thought that progesterone enhances the amount of oxygen in the cells of the brain, thereby increasing mental acuity.

Mood Swings

According to recent research, changes in levels of progesterone have been shown to influence the production and breakdown of brain chemicals that modulate mood. These include the neurotransmitters dopamine, norepinephrine, acetylcholine, and serotonin. Both the peripheral and the central nervous systems have hormone receptors and react to changes in the level of progesterone. Therefore, low progesterone levels will have a direct impact on your ability to maintain a level and balanced mood. It is thought that the ability of progesterone to generate a sense of well-being depends on its brain-related activity.

Stress and Anxiety

As progesterone helps promote a natural calm, a deficiency in this vital hormone can lead to stress and anxiety. In fact, progesterone is sometimes referred to as a natural tranquilizer, as it has a calming and even mildly sedating effect. Taken in high dosages, it has been used as an anesthetic.

It is thought that this calming effect is due to the conversion of progesterone into substances that slow activity at GABA receptors. GABA (gamma aminobutyric acid) is an amino acid that inhibits neuro transmitters (chemicals that relay information from one part of the brain to another) and has a calming effect. While progesterone has a sedating effect on its own, having a balance between estrogen and progesterone levels is crucial for remaining even-tempered under pressure.

Endometrial Cancer

Prevention of endometrial cancer is the primary reason physicians prescribe progesterone during menopause. This became evident several decades ago when the incidence of uterine cancer increased in American women who were prescribed unopposed estrogen. Estrogen use fell into great decline among the menopausal female population until studies showed that combined estrogen therapy could protect women from the development of this cancer. Without the addition of progesterone to an estrogen treatment regimen, the incidence of endometrial (uterine) cancer increases four- to eightfold in women with an intact uterus.

The importance of progesterone therapy in preventing uterine cancer has been emphasized in a number of important medical studies. In one such study, cited in a review article in the *American Family Physician*, 5563 postmenopausal women were followed for nine years.

In women using estrogen alone, the incidence of endometrial cancer was 390.6 cases per 100,000 women per year. In contrast, with combined estrogen and progesterone therapy, the incidence was only 99 cases per 100,000 women per year.

Not only does progesterone confer protection in women using ERT, but it actually appears to protect against the development of endometrial cancer in all postmenopausal women. In the same study, women using no ERT at all were at higher risk than those on progesterone because of their own endogenous estrogen. These women developed 245.5 cases of endometrial cancer per 100,000 women per year.

Not only has the rate of this cancer declined with the use of progesterone, but also those women who develop it tend to do so at a later age.

Heart Disease

There has been quite a bit of controversy surrounding the connection between progesterone and heart disease. Some experts believe that progesterone has no positive effects on the heart, while others claim that it actually increases the "bad" low-density lipoprotein (LDL) cholesterol and decreases the "good" high-density lipoprotein (HDL) cholesterol.

While the experts still debate these issues, what is clear is that the answer lies in the use of natural progesterone versus synthetic progestins. There is strong evidence that natural progesterone causes less fluid retention than progestins, and that the oral, micronized type of natural progesterone may lower blood pressure.

Other research indicates that while synthetic progestins may cause constriction and/or spasms of the blood vessels, natural progesterone has the opposite effect, and actually promotes a widening of the blood vessels — a critical aspect of heart health.

Finally, in a study published in the *Journal of the American Medical Association*. Regimens of estrogen and progesterone (both progestins and oral micronized progesterone) were studied as to their effect on blood lipids. The researchers found that estrogen used in combination with oral micronized progesterone had more beneficial effects on blood lipids than regimens using synthetic progestins.

Osteoporosis

A woman reaches peak bone mass in her early to mid-thirties, after which bone loss slowly begins, accelerating after menopause. A woman can lose 3 to 5 percent of bone mass per year for the first five years after menopause, and 1 to 1.5 percent per year in subsequent years.

Although there has recently been a great deal of media attention on the role of estrogen in bone health, the benefits of progesterone have received far less attention. Nevertheless, as cited in a review article published in *Endocrine* Reviews, a variety of clinical, experimental, and epidemiological data indicate that progesterone plays an important role in bone metabolism

While estrogen does help to prevent osteoporosis by inhibiting calcium loss from the bone and facilitating calcium absorption from the intestinal tract, the addition of progesterone to a treatment regimen may provide even greater benefits. Medical studies have shown that progesterone therapy increases bone mass by promoting new bone formation. Recent research has led to the conclusion that progesterone acts directly to stimulate new bone by attaching to the osteoblast cell receptors — the cells from which new bone tissue is created.

In one study, reported in the *British Medical Journal*, women using combined progesterone and estrogen therapy had a 5 to 6 percent increase in vertebral bone density per year (the gain was slightly greater percentagewise in women on continuous therapy versus cyclical therapy). In another study, published in the *Journal of Gynecological Health*, progesterone and estrogen used in combination increased the bone mineral content significantly, even in women starting the therapy after age sixty. As a result, the addition of progesterone to ERT provides more complete, as well as more effective, treatment for osteoporosis than ERT alone.

A few studies have also suggested that natural progesterone may be effective in protecting women from osteoporosis. John Lee, M.D., a physician in California, has done much research into the use of progesterone to reverse osteoporosis. The results of one of his studies were published in the *International Clinical Nutrition Review*.

Dr. Lee selected 100 patients, Caucasian post-menopausal women between the ages of thirty-eight and eighty-three. The average age was 65.2 at the beginning of the study. The majority of the women had already experienced some loss of height due to osteoporosis.

They were instructed to use conjugated estrogen, 0.3 to 0.625 mg per day for three weeks each month, and progesterone, a 3 percent topical cream, applied daily to the skin for twelve days each month or during the last two weeks of estrogen use. They were also given a dietary and exercise program to follow, plus vitamin and mineral supplements. Alcohol consumption was limited, and no smoking was allowed. The bone health of the women was followed for at least three years.

All the women in the study experienced some degree of progressive increase in bone mineral density, as well as improvement in such clinical symptoms as height stabilization, pain relief, and an increase in physical activity. During the course of the study, there were also no fractures due to osteoporosis per se. These improvements occurred independent of the woman's age.

The women commonly had an increase in the density of vertebral bone of 10 percent in the first six to twelve months of treatment. This increase was purportedly followed by additional yearly increases of 3 to 5 percent. This degree of bone remineralization over a relatively short period of time constitutes an exceptionally good therapeutic response.

I have worked with patients who have been found to have decreased bone density but have refused conventional estrogen/progestin therapy. One such woman, Barbara, chose instead to use natural progesterone cream along with a variety of dietary and plant-based estrogens. She also adopted a vegetarian diet and started performing resistance exercises with weights. Although she had a higher than normal risk of osteoporosis given a 20 percent loss of bone mass by age fifty, she showed a steady improvement in her bone density in the years after initiating this program.

Nerve Damage

Decreased progesterone levels can mean decreased health of your nervous system. Nerves extend throughout your body and are coated with a protective covering called a myelin sheath. These sheaths help protect your nerves from injury caused by trauma and chemical damage, and prevent the electrical impulses from being short-circuited. Myelin is produced by specialized cells called Schwann cells. These cells also produce progesterone, which makes the manufacture of myelin possible.

Besides helping to maintain healthy nerves, progesterone may also be of use in repairing nerve damage.

Animal studies have shown that progesterone levels near the site of a nerve injury are far more concentrated than they normally are in the blood, and when the animals receive additional progesterone, the myelin sheaths surrounding the nerves thicken. This association suggests the possibility that progesterone may one day be useful in the treatment of diseases involving nerve damage, such as multiple sclerosis, which involves a loss of myelin and a resulting impairment of communication functions of the nerves.

7

Testing for Progesterone

Before beginning a progesterone support program or progesterone replacement therapy, it is very helpful to test your own levels of this important hormone. This will help you to best evaluate how effective your treatment program is.

In this chapter, I have included a self-quiz for you to determine if you have symptoms or health conditions that may be caused by a progesterone deficiency. I have also included essential information on laboratory testing for progesterone.

Proper evaluation is very important since low levels of progesterone in women can contribute to a number of health conditions and can negatively affect one's outlook on life, energy level, and emotions.

Checklist: Do You Produce the Progesterone You Need for Peak Performance and Health?

This checklist will give you a preliminary idea of whether you have a deficiency of progesterone. Work through the following checklist (photocopy it if you don't want to write in the book), and refer to it as you read through this section of the chapter. If your responses suggest that your progesterone level is low, you can learn about many ways to support your levels of progesterone in the therapy chapters of this book.

The following checklists can help you determine if you are deficient in progesterone. If you are still menstruating, refer to the first list. If you are in peri-menopause or menopause, then the second list is for you.

Put a check mark beside those statements that are true for you.

Women in Premenopause

If you answer yes to four or more of these questions, you very likely need to increase your progesterone levels.

- o Are you over age 35?
- o Have you gained more than 10 pounds recently?
- o Do you have heavy periods?
- o Do you have irregular periods or spotting?
- o Do you suffer from premenstrual syndrome (PMS), including premenstrual anxiety, irritability and mood swings?
- o Do you suffer from premenstrual fatigue and depression?
- o Do you have difficulty remaining calm under stress?
- o Do you experience premenstrual edema or swollen breasts?
- o Do you get menstrual migraine headaches?
- o Are you retaining fluids?
- o Have you been diagnosed with ovarian cysts?
- o Have you been told you have fibroid tumors?
- o Do you have symptoms of endometriosis?
- o Do you have a decreased interest in sex?
- o Are you experiencing sleep difficulties?
- o Do you have bouts of brain fog—forgetting your friend's first name, where you put your

car keys, or the point of a text you recently studied?

o Do you have difficulty concentrating?
o Have you recently discovered cysts in your breasts?
o Have you been diagnosed with either hyperplasia or endometrial cancer?

Women in Perimenopause or Menopause

If you answer yes to four or more of these questions, you very likely need to increase your progesterone levels.

o Are you age 45 or older?
o Are you in perimenopause?
o Are you in menopause?
o Are you having hot flashes?
o Has your desire for sex faded?
o Do you have difficulty achieving orgasm?
o Is your sleep quality poor?
o Are you often unable to concentrate?
o Are you unable to remain calm under stress?
o Are you frequently tired?
o Are you anxious and irritable?
o Do you forget small details?
o Do your joints and/or muscles ache?
o Do you have osteoporosis?
o Do you have a history of nerve damage?

If you are concerned that either of these checklists sounds like you, you may want to get your hormone levels tested.

Tests to Evaluate the Production of Progesterone

Progesterone levels are commonly assessed through blood testing; however, some testing methods also use saliva, which many women prefer. The level of progesterone measured in the saliva represents about 1 percent of the total blood concentration. This test is thought to be representative of the free versus the bound progesterone within the body. Peak levels with supplemental progesterone use, whether taken orally or as a cream, occur about three hours after use. The lowest levels occur just prior to the next scheduled dose. Readings of progesterone levels help detect luteal insufficiency in the early stages of pregnancy. Progesterone levels are also monitored in women on replacement therapy.

Ranges of salivary progesterone without supplementation in women:

Follicular phase: 0.05 to 0.1 ng/ml
Luteal phase: 0.05 to 0.3 ng/ml

Ranges in saliva with progesterone supplementation:

Transdermal cream users:
> 0.5 ng/ml (peak levels to 100 ng/ml)

Oral micronized progesterone users:
0.05 to 0.5 ng/ml

Ranges of blood progesterone in women:

Menstruating women, luteal phase (mid-cycle):
7 to 28 ng/ml

Normal, untreated, postmenopausal women:
0.03 to 0.3 ng/ml

After three months' treatment with transdermal progesterone: 3 to 4 ng/ml

In addition to blood testing, there are also saliva tests for female hormones. Unlike blood tests, saliva tests are non-invasive (no needle sticks!) and highly accurate. These tests can take the guesswork out of making a proper diagnosis and make it possible to design individualized treatment that delivers maximum benefits with minimum risk of side effects.

Best of all, saliva hormone testing is accessible. Even physicians who still don't routinely order saliva hormone testing will usually write an order when a patient requests it. You can even order a limited saliva hormone test kit on your own directly from a laboratory, without a doctor's order. (See below for specific recommendations.)

Like blood, saliva closely mirrors hormone levels in your body's tissues. However, saliva is a particularly accurate indicator of free (unbound) hormone levels. This is the key, as only free hormones are active, meaning that they can affect the hormone-sensitive tissues in your breasts, brain, heart, and uterus. Saliva testing therefore provides a superior measure of the levels of hormones that actually affect vital body systems, mood, tissue levels of sodium and fluid, and many other important functions.

Additionally, blood testing only provides a one time "snapshot" of hormone levels, whereas saliva testing provides a dynamic picture of hormonal ebb and flow over an entire menstrual cycle. In fact, 11 samples are collected during the month, all at the same time of day, and then sent to a laboratory. The lab then measures and charts your progesterone levels. These results are compared to normal patterns.

Getting Tested

If you think saliva hormone testing is right for you, consider consulting your physician. Having your doctor order the test has two advantages: The profile is more extensive, and your insurance may cover the cost. Several laboratories perform the test; in the event your physician does not have a preference, I recommend Genova Diagnostic (gdx.net or 800-522-4762), as well as ZRT Laboratory (zrtlab.com or 866-600-1636). If your doctor doesn't order the test, or you simply want insight to help you develop your own self-care regimen, you can order a test kit from several sources. Aeron Laboratories has a wonderful Life Cycles saliva test kit (aeron.com or 800-631-7900).

Progesterone levels are also commonly assessed with blood testing. If you opt for saliva testing, keep in mind that the level of progesterone measured in your saliva represents about one percent of the total blood concentration.

This test is thought to be representative of the free versus the bound progesterone within your body. Peak levels with supplemental progesterone use, whether taken orally or as a cream, occur about three hours after use. The lowest levels occur just prior to the next scheduled dose. Readings of progesterone levels help detect luteal insufficiency in the early stages of pregnancy. Progesterone levels are also monitored in women on replacement therapy.

Ranges of salivary progesterone without supplementation:

Follicular phase: < 0.1 ng/ml*
Luteal phase: 0.1 to 0.5 ng/ml*

Ranges in saliva with progesterone supplementation:

Transdermal cream users: 1.0 to 10 ng/ml*
Oral micronized progesterone users:
0.1 to 0.5 ng/ml*

Ranges of blood progesterone:

Menstruating women, luteal phase (mid-cycle):
5 to 20 ng/ml *
Normal, untreated, postmenopausal women:
< 1.0 ng/ml**

If your results indicate that you are deficient in progesterone (or if you scored high on the checklist), you are far from alone. I have treated thousands of women with decreased levels of this hormone. Let's take a look at how you can replenish your progesterone levels safely and effectively.

* figures from Aeron Biotechnology

** figures from MedlinePlus (a service of the US National Library of Medicine and the National Institutes of Health)

8

Restoring Your Own Progesterone

Throughout my years in the field of women's health, I've worked with a number of substances that have been very useful in helping women increase their own progesterone production. I have had wonderful success over the years using these safe, gentle, effective nutritional and other lifestyle-related therapies to accomplish this goal. Many of my patients have had great results and have been thrilled with the benefits.

My program is a better, safer way to help you navigate through the progesterone deficiency related to premenopause, as well as perimenopause and menopause, with greatly diminished symptoms. In the case of premenopause-related conditions, my program has helped women avoid surgical procedures like hysterectomies, as well as reduce or eliminate the need to use medications that can cause very severe side effects, and treat conditions such as uterine fibroids, endometriosis, and severe PMS.

With my program, you'll use nutrients to help you stimulate progesterone production at the nervous system level as well as in the ovaries. You'll also learn how supplemental, natural, biochemically identical progesterone can help increase levels of this vital hormone.

Stimulate Your Own Progesterone Production

To increase progesterone production, it is necessary to stimulate and support ovulation. This can be done on two levels—through the central nervous system or via the ovaries.

While women are surprised to learn that you can increase progesterone production through the brain or central nervous system, the truth is that all hormone production begins in the brain.

Support Progesterone Production Through Brain Balance

There are three key types of brain chemicals: neuropeptides, neurohormones, and neurotransmitters. All of these chemicals affect our production of female hormones and our hormonal balance, including progesterone production.

Neuropeptides are responsible for the cell-to-cell communication system in your body. A peptide is a short chain of amino acids connected together, and a neuropeptide is a peptide found in neural tissue. Neuropeptides are widespread in the central and peripheral nervous systems and different neuropeptides have different excitatory or inhibitory actions.

Neuropeptides control such a diverse array of functions in the body. When they work together properly, the wonderful results in your body include elevated mood and other positive behaviors and emotions, stronger bones, better resistance to disease, glowing skin, and boosted metabolism. Conversely, if your neuropeptides function abnormally, the result can be an increased tendency towards neurological and mental disorders such as Alzheimer's disease, epilepsy, and schizophrenia.

There are several types of neuropeptides. Some of the most common include endorphins and beta-endorphins. Endorphins are opiod peptides, meaning they have morphine-like effects within the body. They produce feelings of well-being and euphoria, and a rush of endorphins can lead to feelings of exhilaration brought on by pain, danger, or stress. Endorphins also may also play a role in memory, sexual activity, and body temperature. Beta-endorphins are another form of opiod peptides, but they are stronger than endorphins. They are composed of 31 amino acids and work in the body by numbing pain, increasing relaxation, and promoting a general feeling of well-being.

While there are many, many hormones and hormonal interactions that occur in the brain and body, the most widely known neurohormone is melatonin.

Neurotransmitters are naturally occurring chemicals that relay electrical messages between nerve cells throughout your body. While all three types of neurochemicals are important for hormone and overall health, neurotransmitters are particularly important for the production of sex hormones.

In the aggregate, all three types of neurochemicals help to regulate the brain's endocrine glands, specifically the hypothalamus and pituitary gland. The hypothalamus is the master endocrine gland contained within your brain that regulates your production of sex hormones. This gland produces a precursor hormone called gonadotropin releasing hormone (GnRH). When it is released, it travels to your anterior pituitary gland, where it stimulates the secretion of the follicle stimulating (FSH) and luteinizing hormones (LH).

These hormones then travel to the adrenals and ovaries, where they stimulate the production of estrogen, progesterone, and testosterone. In women with decreased levels of progesterone, the production of LH needed to trigger ovulation may not proceed in a healthy fashion.

In order to keep this whole process working smoothly, LH and FSH need to be triggered by a balanced mixture of the key neurotransmitters necessary to produce these hormones. The production of these vital chemicals is synthesized from certain amino acids, vitamins, and minerals that must be obtained through your diet or from supplementation.

First and foremost, the neurotransmitters norepinephrine, epinephrine, dopamine, and serotonin regulate the hypothalamus' release of GnRH. Without proper production and balance of these neurotransmitters, you cannot have proper balance of the sex hormones, including progesterone. This process is supported by precursor amino acids such as tyrosine, phenylalanine, and 5-HTP.

To understand this more fully, let's take a more detailed look at neurotransmitters in action.

Neurotransmitters: The Hormone Messengers

There are two crucial neurotransmitter pathways that help to support your overall health and well-being. The first leads to the production of the inhibitory neurotransmitter serotonin, while the second leads to the production of the excitatory neurotransmitters dopamine, norepinephrine, and epinephrine.

Generally speaking, the inhibitory neurotransmitters quiet down the processes of your body, while the excitatory neurotransmitters speed them up. Thus, the brain chemicals produced through these two pathways oppose and complement one another. Within your brain, serotonin often inhibits the firing of neurons, which dampens many of your behaviors. In fact, serotonin acts as a kind of chemical restraint system.

Of all your body's chemicals, serotonin has one of the most widespread effects on the brain and physiology. It plays a key role in regulating temperature, blood pressure, blood clotting, immunity, pain, digestion, sleep, and biorhythms. Along with another inhibitory neurotransmitters GABA (gamma-aminobutyric acid) and taurine, serotonin also produces a relaxing effect on your mood. Glutamate is another important excitatory neurotransmitter, though it is not part of the pathway.

Dopamine, norepinephrine, and epinephrine make up the excitatory neurotransmitter pathway. Unlike serotonin, which has a relaxing effect on your energy and behavior, excitatory neurotransmitters energize and elevate your mood. In addition to their powerful anti-depressant effects, they support alertness, optimism, motivation, zest for life, and sex drive. Plus, the excitatory neurotransmitters are particularly important for the production of progesterone.

In order to ensure that you have adequate neuro-transmitter levels for healthy hormone production, you need to supplement with key amino acids, vitamins, and minerals. All neurotransmitters are produced from amino acids found in the protein that you eat. The essential amino acid tryptophan is initially converted into an intermediary substance called 5-hydroxytryptophan (5-HTP), which is then converted into serotonin.

While tryptophan is available as a supplement and is abundant in turkey, pumpkin seeds, and almonds, I've found that 5-HTP is a more effective and reliable option for boosting your neurotransmitter prod-uction. Numerous double-blind studies have shown that 5-HTP is as effective as many of the more com-mon anti-depressant drugs and is associated with fewer and much milder side effects. In addition to increasing serotonin levels, 5-HTP triggers an increase in endorphins and other neurotransmitters that are often low in cases of depression.

Do You Have a Neurotransmitter Imbalance?

If you experience any of the following symptoms on an ongoing, consistent basis, you may have a neuro-transmitter imbalance.

Low Inhibitory Neurotransmitters

- PMS
- Migraine headaches
- Chronic pain
- Irritable bowel syndrome
- Mood swings, irritability
- Anxiety
- Food cravings, binge eating
- Sleep apnea
- Fibromyalgia
- Increased infections
- Insomnia, poor sleep quality

Low Excitatory Neurotransmitters

- Depression
- Fatigue
- Low thyroid function
- High stress levels
- Weight gain, difficulty losing weight
- Cold hands and feet
- Mental sluggishness
- Low libido
- Irregular menstruation, heavy bleeding

The excitatory neurotransmitters are derived from tyrosine, an amino acid produced from phenylalanine, another amino acid. A variety of vitamins and minerals, such as vitamin C, vitamin B6, and magnesium, act as co-factors and are necessary for the conversion of these amino acids into neurotransmitters.

To maintain proper serotonin levels, it is helpful to take 50-100 mg of 5-HTP per day, preferably at bedtime. You may want to start as low as 50 mg and increase as necessary. If needed during the day, use carefully, as too much serotonin can interfere with your ability to drive or concentrate.

To maintain optimum dopamine levels, take 500-1,000 mg of tyrosine per day. Be sure to take in divided doses, half in the morning and half in the afternoon. Do not take in the evening, as it may interfere with sleep.

As I recommend with all nutritional supplements, you should start at the lower to more moderate dosage, such as 500 mg a day of tyrosine and 50 mg a day of 5-HTP. Stay on this dosage for two weeks. If you don't notice a reduction in your symptoms, gradually increase the dosage by 500 mg for tyrosine and 50 mg for 5-HTP every two weeks until you have either noticed a reduction in your symptoms or have reached the maximum dosages. I generally don't recommend going over 1,000 mg a day of tyrosine, although you may find that you need as much as 100-200 mg of 5-HTP once or even several times a day.

Additionally, be sure to use a high potency multi vitamin/mineral nutritional supplement so that you are taking in all of the co-factors needed to produce neurotransmitters. These include vitamin C, vitamin B6, folic acid, niacin, magnesium, and copper.

Note: I strongly advise that you undertake a program to restore and properly balance your neurotransmitter levels under the care of a complementary physician, naturopath, or nutritionist. You should also have your neurotransmitter levels tested regularly, as dosage needs vary from woman to woman.

Test Your Neurotransmitter Levels

State-of-the-art neurotransmitter testing is currently available and can accurately pinpoint your exact levels of these essential brain chemicals. Neuro-Science, Inc., (888-342-7272 or neurorelief.com) is a leader in the development of neurotransmitter testing. They have developed sensitive testing for these neurochemicals that can be done through your urine. The test is simple to do, non-invasive, and can be done in the privacy of your own home. In addition to NeuroScience, there are many other similar laboratories that offer neurotransmitter testing.

I would strongly recommend that you consider such testing if you suspect that you suffer from a moderate to severe neurotransmitter deficiency. Your health care provider will need to order these tests for you.

Herbs That Benefit Neurotransmitter Production and Progesterone

In addition to creating proper neurotransmitter balance through the use of amino acids derived from your diet, with the help of key vitamins and minerals, there are several other types of nutrients that can help to keep your endocrine glands and precursor hormones functioning properly. My particular favorites include vitex (chaste tree berry), maca, and glandulars.

Vitex (Chaste Tree Berry)

Vitex is an herb native to the Mediterranean area. It works at the hypothalamic and pituitary levels. Specifically, it aids in the production of LH to trigger ovulation, thereby promoting progesterone production.

One interesting study found that vitex helps restore menstruation by increasing progesterone levels. Researchers gave vitex extract to 20 women who had either abnormal or non-existent menstruation. After six months, 15 of the women were available for evaluation. Lab tests revealed that 10 of the 15 women had a return of their menstrual cycles, as well as increased levels of both progesterone and LH.

A similar study found that eight women with abnormally low progesterone levels who were given vitex every day for three months also enjoyed increased progesterone levels. In fact, two of the women became pregnant!

Vitex has also been shown to hinder the release of prolactin, a hormone closely related to human growth hormone, which plays a critical role in lactation. If there is too much prolactin in your system, secretion of LH is disturbed, which in turn can disrupt ovulation, and therefore progesterone production.

Several studies have proven vitex's ability to reduce prolactin levels. One double-blind, placebo-controlled study examined 52 women with luteal phase problems due to increased prolactin levels. They were given 20 mg of vitex a day for three months. At the end of the treatment period, prolactin levels had been significantly reduced.

A study from *Experimental and Clinical Endocrinology* suggests that vitex works to decrease prolactin by binding to dopamine receptors, which in turn thwart the secretion of prolactin. Interestingly, the researchers found that while prolactin secretion was inhibited, gonadotropin secretion (which leads to FSH and LH secretion) remained unaffected.

Research from several German peer-reviewed publications confirms this finding. For example, the *International Journal of Gynecology & Obstetrics*, and *Hormone and Metabolic Research* have both found that vitex appears to block prolactin secretion by binding to dopamine receptors. However, much research still needs to be done in this area.

To increase progesterone levels and decrease prolactin, I suggest taking 140-275 mg of a standardized extract of vitex (chaste tree berry) every day. Chaste tree berry works slowly, so it may take three or four months before you start to see its full benefit.

Maca

Maca — referred to as either Lepidium peruvianum or Lepidium meyenii — is one of the most traditionally used and valued Peruvian herbs, due in large part to its rich nutrient concentration. This malty, butterscotch-flavored root contains a number of minerals, vitamins, fatty acids, plant sterols, amino acids, and alkaloids, among other phytonutrients. In terms of minerals, calcium makes up 10 percent of maca's mineral content. Magnesium, phosphorus, and potassium are also present in significant amounts. Maca also contains a number of vitamins and amino acids, including B1, B2, B12, vitamin C, vitamin E, and quercetin, as well as arginine, lysine, tryptophan, tyrosine, and phenylalanine.

German and American researchers begin studying Peruvian botanicals in the 1960's and 1980's. They quickly discovered that maca has many health benefits, including relieving menopausal symptoms; stimulating and regulating the endocrine system (adrenals, thyroid, ovaries, and testes); increasing energy, stamina, and endurance; regulating and normalizing menstrual cycles; and balancing hormone levels.

Maca appears to act as a central nervous system stimulant, at the level of the hypothalamus and pituitary gland. It works to stimulate hormone production, which is critical to regulate so much of a woman's physiology. It also operates as an adaptogenic herb to help regulate hormones produced by the endocrine glands. It does this by stimulating your ovaries and adrenals to produce the hormones you need, in the levels that you need them.

This was shown in a study published in the *Journal of Veterinary Medical Science*. Researchers tested the effects of maca on mouse sex hormones. They found that progesterone and testosterone levels increased significantly in the mice that received the maca.

A traditional dosage of maca is 2-10 grams a day. However, dosages are unique to each woman, so you will need to determine which dosage works for you. There have been no acute toxic effects of maca, even at very high doses. In fact, many Peruvians eat it every day! Note: If you are sensitive or allergic to herbs, you may want to use maca cautiously. In any event, I suggest starting with the low end of the recommended dosage, as too much can cause increased hot flashes, breast tenderness, or headache. It is also recommended that you avoid maca if you have a hormone-related cancer (due to lack of formal studies), liver disease, if you are pregnant or nursing, or if you are currently taking conventional HRT.

Glandular Therapy

Glandular therapy involves the use of purified extracts from the secretory endocrine glands of animals. Most commonly, extracts are drawn from the thyroid and adrenal glands, as well as the thymus, pituitary, pancreas, and ovaries. Most extracts come from cows (bovine glandulars), with the exception of pancreatic glandular preparations usually drawn from sheep.

There are four common ways to extract glandulars. The first involves quick-freezing the material, washing it with a potent solvent to remove fatty tissues, distilling the solvent out, drying it, and then grinding it into a fine powder that is then encapsulated or pressed into tablets.

The second mixes freshly crushed material with salt and water that also removes fatty tissues. It is then dried and ground into a fine powder to be placed in capsules or made into tablets.

In the third method, the glandular material is freeze-dried, then placed into a vacuum chamber to remove the water. It is then encapsulated. However, with this method, fatty tissues remain.

The final method uses plant and animal enzymes to partially "digest" the material. It is then passed through a filter that separates out the fat-soluble molecules. The remaining material is then freeze-dried. This method seems to be quite effective. Due to the "predigestion," all biologically active substances remain intact and can be used therapeutically to support and restore your body's endocrine glands. Healthier endocrine glands are more likely to have healthier hormone production and to be more balanced.

In the past, most experts believed that glandulars could not be effective because the intestinal lining of a healthy person was impenetrable, and that proteins and large peptides could not breach its barrier. However, recent evidence has shown that large macromolecules can and do pass completely intact from the intestinal tract into the bloodstream. In fact, there's further evidence to suggest that your body is able to determine which molecules it needs to absorb whole, and which can be broken down.

Both animal and human studies alike have proven this theory. In some cases, several whole proteins taken orally, including critical enzymes, have been shown to be absorbed intact into the bloodstream. Additionally, many smaller proteins and numerous hormones have also been found to be absorbed intact into the bloodstream, including thyroid, cortisone, and even insulin.

In essence, it means that the active properties of the glandulars stay active and intact, and are not destroyed in the digestive process. This is key to the success of glandular therapy, and explains why they clearly help to restore hormone function by supporting the health of your endocrine glands themselves.

There are multi- and single-glandular systems available from companies like Standard Process—a leader in the field. However, they do require a prescription from a health care practitioner. Other good products are also available in health food stores and should be used as part of a nutritional program to support healthy menstruation.

Examples of widely used and accepted glandulars involve the thyroid and the adrenals. Natural thyroid medications such as Armour Thyroid, Naturthyroid, and Bio-Thyroid have been the preference of complementary physicians for decades. Unlike many of the commonly prescribed brands of thyroid therapy that only replace a synthetic form of T4, these natural thyroid replacements contain the whole animal-derived thyroid gland, including T3 and T4. This is a significant difference. T3 is more physiologically active than T4, and is critical in regulating normal growth and energy metabolism. Without the use of glandulars, this type of natural thyroid replacement wouldn't be possible. However, the thyroid glandulars sold in the health food stores have the hormone removed and are used to support the function of your own gland.

Adrenal glandular preparations are even more common. With the stress epidemic in this country, the majority of Americans are walking around with depressed adrenal function. This can also manifest as fatigue, susceptibility to infection, allergies, and infection.

Fortunately, whole adrenal extracts have been shown to possess cortisone-like properties that help treat asthma, eczema, rheumatoid arthritis, and even psoriasis. They have also been found to help restore the health and function of comprised adrenal glands. In one research study, eight women suffering from morning sickness (nausea and vomiting) who took oral adrenal cortex extract found relief within four days. A similar study gave both injected and oral adrenal cortex extract to 202 women also suffering from morning sickness. More than 85 percent of the women completely overcame their nausea and vomiting or showed significant improvement.

Another study looked at the use of adrenal glandulars to treat patients with chronic fatigue and immune dysfunction syndrome (CFIDS), as well as fibromyalgia. Researchers found that 5-13 mg of an adrenal glandular preparation significantly reduced pain and discomfort. Moreover, after six to 18 months, many of the patients were able to reduce and eventually discontinue treatment, while still enjoying relief.

Clearly, glandulars work. To help support healthy progesterone levels, I suggest taking a good multi-glandular or single glandular product from a company like Standard Process. These could include glandulars such as hypothalamus, pituitary, ovary, adrenal, and thyroid, depending on the specific needs of each individual woman. I also highly recommend that you consider taking a whole brain glandular, if appropriate. To further support your adrenal function, I recommend taking 1,000-3,000 mg of a mineral-buffered vitamin C each day with a meal, 25-100 mg of a vitamin B complex a day, and an additional 250 mg of B5 (pantothenic acid) twice a day.

While stimulating progesterone production origin-ates in your central nervous system, you also need to support progesterone production in your ovaries.

Support Progesterone Production Through Ovarian Balance

Like estrogen and testosterone, progesterone is also produced by your ovaries, making it critical that you keep your ovaries functioning at their optimal level. To do this, I highly recommend using the following key nutrients: lutein, beta-carotene, and essential fatty acids.

Lutein

Lutein is a carotenoid with powerful antioxidant properties. As you can likely determine from its name, lutein plays a major role in the luteal phase, the time from ovulation to menstruation when the luteinizing hormone (LH) is produced.

While estrogen levels are rising from menstruation through ovulation, LH, which is produced by the pituitary gland, is needed to trigger ovulation. After ovulation, the follicle that contained the egg that was expelled from the ovary during ovulation is then converted into a new structure called the corpus luteum. Lutein is abundant in the corpus luteum and provides it with its distinctive yellow color.

The purpose of the corpus luteum is to switch from the estrogen production, which predominates during the first half of the menstrual cycle (days one to 14) to the production of progesterone and estrogen during the second half of your cycle (days 15 to 28). This is called the luteinizing process. During this time, lutein begins to accumulate in these key cells, and the effectiveness of the luteinizing process may be due, in part, to the amount of lutein found there. To ensure that you have adequate lutein levels to support normal development of the corpus luteum, I suggest supplementing with 6-12 mg of lutein a day.

Beta-Carotene

Beta-carotene is the plant-based, water-soluble precursor to vitamin A. Like lutein, beta-carotene is abundant in the ovaries, and is found in very high concentrations in the corpus luteum. Some research even suggests that a proper balance between carotene and the retinal form of vitamin A is necessary for proper luteal function.

Researchers have been aware of the reproductive benefits of beta-carotene for more than a century. For example, cows whose diets were deficient in beta-carotene experienced delayed ovulation, decreased progesterone levels, and an increased prevalence of ovarian cysts, as well as cystic mastitis (breast cysts). Both conditions are typically found in women who are progesterone deficient.

Studies have also determined that high doses of vitamin A can help reverse one form of benign breast disease. In a study from *Preventative Medicine*, researchers gave 150,000 IU of vitamin A to 12 women with fibrocystic breasts. After three months, more than half the women reported complete or partial remission of the cysts. While I would never suggest that women take this high a dose of vitamin A for fear of toxicity, I believe that beta-carotene would have a similar effect.

To ensure that you have adequate amounts of vitamin A (as beta-carotene) in your system, I suggest taking 25,000-50,000 IU of beta-carotene a day.

Essential Fatty Acids

Essential fatty acids (EFAs) are health-promoting nutrients that your body needs to perform a whole range of functions. There are two main groups of EFAs: omega-3s and omega-6s. The most common are linoleic acid (omega-6), linolenic acid (omega-3), and the omega-3 fatty acids eicosapentaenoic acid (EPA) and docosahexaenoic acid (DHA).

Your body converts EFAs into series 1 and 3 prostaglandins, potent hormone-like substances with a wide range of benefits that are essential for good reproductive health. Among other things, these prostaglandins help to promote more frequent ovulation at mid-cycle. Since prostaglandins are necessary for the rupture of the follicle, which allows the egg to be extruded from the ovary at mid-cycle, this is a critical step for progesterone production to occur during the second half of the cycle.

The two best sources of EFAs are flaxseed and fish oil. In the case of flaxseed, both the oil and the ground meal are rich in EFAs. Plus, flax has been proven to support progesterone production. Researchers at the University of Minnesota tested 18 women with normal menstrual cycles. During three cycles, the women ate as they normally would. They then added 10 grams of ground flaxseed per day to their diet for an additional three cycles. The women who ate flaxseed had more ovulatory cycles than the women who did not.

In addition, ground flaxseed was found to improve the estrogen-to-progesterone ratio, favoring the levels of progesterone within the body. The researchers felt that this was due to the lignans contained in the flaxseed, although I feel strongly that the flaxseed oil was also very beneficial in this regard, as it is also converted into prostaglandins, which is needed to allow ovulation to occur. To promote progesterone production, I suggest taking 1-2 tablespoons of flaxseed oil or 4-6 tablespoons of ground flaxseed per day.

If you do not like flaxseed or cannot tolerate it, you may prefer to get your EFAs through fish oil. In addition to also promoting progesterone production and helping to regulate the menstrual cycle, fish oil is extremely beneficial for easing menstrual cramps, endometriosis, and breast cysts due to its anti-inflammatory benefits. If fish oil is your preference, I suggest taking 3-6 capsules that contain at least 300 mg DHA and 200 mg EPA every day.

9

Supplement with Bioidentical Progesterone

For many women, supplementing with bioidentical progesterone can be tremendously helpful in restoring a healthy balance between the level of estrogen and progesterone within the body. Natural, bioidentical progesterone can also relieve the symptoms of issues like PMS, menopause, endometrial hyperplasia and many other conditions with little to no negative side effects. I have recommended bioidentical progesterone to many patients over the years and have been incredibly pleased with the positive results. Many of my patients have been absolutely thrilled by how much better they felt once they started to use progesterone therapy.

In discussing progesterone replacement therapy, I do want to clear up any misunderstanding of what the term "natural" means. The progesterone used in replacement therapy today, whether described as synthetic or natural, is all produced by commercial laboratories.

The terms natural and synthetic refer to the actual structure of the progesterone molecule. Progesterone that is natural has the same structure as the hormone the body produces. In contrast, while synthetic progesterone has somewhat the same function as the progesterone produced by the body, its structure also differs. In the United States, most prescriptions given to patients by their physician are for the synthetic form, called a progestin. The most common progestin is Provera, or medroxyprogesterone.

Progesterone became an important topic for women in the 1970's when its important role in preventing endometrial cancer in postmenopausal women on estrogen replacement therapy (ERT) was discovered. In one study, cited in a review article in the *American Family Physician*, 5,563 postmenopausal women were followed for nine years. In women using estrogen alone, the incidence of endometrial cancer was 390.6 cases per 100,000 women per year. In contrast, with combined estrogen and progesterone therapy, the incidence was only 99 cases per 100,000 women per year.

Not only does progesterone confer protection in women using estrogen replacement therapy, but it actually appears to protect against the development of endometrial cancer in all postmenopausal women. In the same study, women using no estrogen therapy at all were at higher risk than those on progesterone because of their own endogenous estrogen. These women developed 245.5 cases of endometrial cancer per 100,000 women per year. Not only has the rate of this cancer declined with the use of progesterone, but also those women who develop it tend to do so at a later age. After this and other similar studies, progesterone therapy rapidly became part of the standard hormonal regimen for postmenopausal women who still had their uterus intact.

Before the 1980's, all progesterone therapy had to be administered by injection in the doctor's office. The development of oral progesterone-like chemicals made this hormone much more readily available. Initially, a synthetic type of progesterone was combined with estrogen in birth control pills for younger women as well as hormone replacement therapy for women suffering from menopause related symptoms.

Fortunately, natural progesterone became available in the early 1980s but initially only as a rectal or vaginal suppository. Although many women found the use of natural progesterone to be helpful, using it as a suppository was messy, since it tended to leak from the rectum or vagina. Synthetic progestin remained the preferred form because it was easy to take as a pill and also more absorbable.

However, natural progesterone was subsequently developed in a topical form that can be rubbed into the skin and is available over-the-counter. It is also prescribed by physicians in a micronized form (pulverized into tiny particles) called Prometrium that is readily absorbed and can be taken orally. This is much more convenient for many women and easier and less messy to use. Today, many women prefer using natural progesterone, as it produces fewer side effects than the synthetic progestins.

It's important to thoroughly understand the difference between synthetic and natural progesterone, since, as I already mentioned, they do not have the same chemical structure and do not behave the same biologically. They also differ in their benefits and side effects. Let's take a more in-depth look at the two main progesterone replacements available — progestins and natural, bioidentical progesterone.

Synthetic Progestins

The first chemical (or synthetic) progestin was developed in the early 1950's by Mexican chemist Luis Miramontes. Over the last half century, it has continued to gain acceptance in the conventional medical community and is still commonly prescribed by many mainstream physicians.

Progestins have been traditionally used during the transition into menopause. Perimenopausal women may produce too much estrogen without ovulating, which can cause heavy periods lasting as long as 10 to 12 days, or even longer. Taking progestins alone can help prevent erratic heavy periods. Progestins also help prevent the heavy buildup of endometrial lining by making sure that the lining is completely shed each month. By promoting a regular menstrual period each month, the use of progestins can also help reduce the number of endometrial biopsies a woman's physician needs to perform.

Routes of Administration and Dosages

Oral tablets of synthetic progesterone are the most widely prescribed form of progesterone. To regulate the menstrual cycle, only small doses of progestins, usually 5 to 10 mg, are needed. Some women require slightly higher or lower doses. Progestins are often used 10 to 13 days per month. The most commonly used brand of progestins is Provera (Upjohn). Norlutate (Parke-Davis) is also frequently prescribed, but it may cause side effects similar to those of androgens, such as oily skin and acne. A third progestin currently on the market is Amen (Carnick).

Physicians have also used progestins for many years as part of a conventional HRT regimen that is prescribed by most doctors. This is most often used by women who are menopausal, or those who have had surgically induced menopause, but still have their ovaries. Progestins can even be used alone by women who cannot take (or cannot tolerate) estrogen. Although it is not as effective as estrogen for reducing the severity of hot flashes, many women can still find some relief with a progestin. In fact, one study found that an injectable progestin (Depo-Provera) relieved hot flashes in nearly 90 percent of women.

However, the use of progestins has many drawbacks. In addition to increased risk of breast cancer and heart disease, some women taking progestins experience debilitating side effects. These often include abnormal bleeding, fatigue, headaches, depression and mood changes, bloating, breast tenderness and enlargement, vaginal dryness, and increased appetite. If any of these occur, physicians will often reduce the dosage.

Side Effects

Some women taking progestins experience side effects that include fatigue, headaches, depression and mood changes, bloating, breast tenderness and enlargement, and increased appetite. If any of these occur, dosages should be decreased to as low as 1.25 mg per day.

Progestins can also cause more serious problems, such as an increased risk of heart disease. A study published in the *Journal of the American College of Cardiology* looked at monkeys that were made vulnerable to coronary spasms. The researchers treated the monkeys with estrogen, and this tendency was completely reversed. Then six monkeys were given a combined treatment of estrogen plus progesterone, and six others estrogen plus progestins. The progestin treatment resulted in coronary-artery spasms in all the monkeys, while those receiving natural progesterone had no spasms.

In human trials, progestins (especially when combined with synthetic estrogen) also prove to be problematic. In the PEPI (Postmenopausal Estrogen-Progestin Intervention) trial study, all of the women who took estrogen alone, estrogen and the progestin medroxyprogesterone (Provera), or estrogen with micronized (oral) progesterone experienced increases in their C-reactive protein levels. C-reactive protein, an indicator of inflammation, is now known to be a very strong predictor of future heart attacks, superior to LDL or HDL levels. Similarly, in the Heart and Estrogen/Progestin Replacement Study (HERS) trial, women taking a synthetic estrogen/progestin combination suffered significantly more heart attacks and other heart problems than those receiving a placebo.

Worse yet, progestins also appear to lower the "good" HDL cholesterol associated with a lower risk of heart disease, though the results of some studies do conflict with this. In the PEPI trials, women taking estrogen and progestins had lower HDL levels, while women on estrogen and natural, biochemically identical progesterone maintained higher levels of HDL.

There is also evidence that progestins may have a harmful effect on various systems of the body if taken over a long period, and can increase the risk of birth defects if taken during the first four months of pregnancy.

Natural Progesterone

In my opinion, any woman considering taking progesterone for its performance, as well as health benefits, should consider using natural progesterone rather than the progestins. In my own clinical practice, I initially prescribed it for my PMS patients, but also found that it was useful for problems related to estrogen dominance, as well as menopause.

Natural (or biochemically identical) progesterone is produced from dioscorea, the active component of the Mexican wild yam—as are pregnenolone and DHEA. It can also be manufactured from soybeans. In either case, the resultant hormone has the same chemical structure and range of activity as the progesterone made by your body.

Natural progesterone appears to confer an equal amount of protection against uterine cancer and functions as a diuretic and an anti-anxiety treatment. It can also stimulate libido, help prevent and treat fibrocystic breast disease, regulate thyroid hormone activity, stabilize blood sugar levels, and assist in normal blood clotting. Plus, natural progesterone is essential for the production of cortisone in the adrenal cortex, and helps convert fat to energy.

Beyond all these benefits, natural progesterone also plays an important role in the prevention and reversal of osteoporosis. In a study conducted by Dr. John Lee, published in *Medical Hypotheses*, 100 postmenopausal women were treated with natural progesterone for a minimum of three years. Without treatment, these women would have had an expected bone loss of 4.5 percent. However, the bone density of the women was found to increase-10 percent in the first year on average, followed by a yearly increase of 3 to 5 percent thereafter.

When natural progesterone is taken in normally prescribed amounts (see next page), there are no known side effects. However, very high doses can cause drowsiness, due to its sedative effect on the brain, and huge doses of the hormone can act as an anesthetic or cause a person to feel drunk. During the beginning stages of supplementing with progest- erone, a woman may have symptoms of estrogen dominance. This happens because progesterone can increase the sensitivity of estrogen receptor sites. However, this sensitivity will disappear after a few weeks.

Using Natural Progesterone

Women of all ages (from their 30's on up) are currently using natural progesterone cream, which is now available in many health food stores and does not require a doctor's prescription (although the other forms of natural progesterone do require a prescription). Natural progesterone can be taken in oral micronized form or as a skin cream, rectal or vaginal suppository, or sublingual drops. Be sure to check the label of any product that you buy to make sure it truly contains pharmaceutical-grade, natural progesterone in therapeutic doses. There are a number of brands on the market, such as Emerita Pro-Gest Cream.

Oral Micronized Progesterone

Initially, natural progesterone could not be taken orally because it was destroyed during digestion and never reached the bloodstream. However, a micronized form of progesterone is now available that is protected from destruction by stomach acid and enzymes and can be absorbed and used by the body.

One study published in the *British Medical Journal* followed 23 women for four months. Each woman received 300 mg of oral progesterone daily for two continuous months. Those women receiving treatment had a clear improvement in concentration. Similar increases in mental acuity and the ability to remain focused on a subject have also been found in premenopausal and postmenopausal women.

Research has shown that oral progesterone can also reduce blood pressure. In a study also published in the *British Medical Journal*, researchers gave post-menopausal women and older men 200, 400, or 600 mg of oral progesterone or a placebo every day for two weeks. Those taking the progesterone enjoyed a significant decrease in their systolic blood pressure (the top number), as compared to the placebo group. In fact, participants who took 600 mg lowered their systolic blood pressure by about 19.7 mm Hg and their diastolic blood pressure (the bottom number) by about 9.6 mm Hg.

In menopausal women, dosages of 100-200 mg of natural, oral progesterone (Prometrium) taken daily can be effective, although the dose can vary in either direction. You need these high doses, as 85-90 percent of the amount consumed will be metabolized by the liver soon after it has been ingested. Like the synthetic progestins, perimenopausal women should use oral micronized progesterone 10-13 days per month. If you are in menopause, most physicians advise using it every day. Prometrium must be prescribed by a physician, unlike progesterone cream, which can be purchased over-the-counter.

Skin Cream

Progesterone cream is getting rave reviews from women and researchers alike. According to a double-blind, randomized, placebo-controlled study from *Obstetrics & Gynecology*, transdermal progesterone cream relieved menopausal vasomotor symptoms.

Researchers tested 90 postmenopausal women who were within five years of menopause and had not used any hormones for at least 12 months prior to the study. The women were tested for follicle-stimulating hormone levels; bone mineral density of the lumbar spine and hip; cholesterol levels; LDL, HDL, and triglyceride levels, and thyroid-stimulating hormone levels. All of the tests were repeated after one year. During that time, each woman kept a log of the number and severity of hot flashes.

The women were divided into two groups. In the first group, 43 of the women used 1/4 teaspoon (20 mg) of progesterone cream a day, regularly rotating the appli-cation on their arm, breasts, or thighs. The other 47 women used a placebo. Of the women using the progesterone cream, 83 percent enjoyed fewer hot flashes, as compared to just 19 percent in the placebo group.

This finding was also confirmed by a study reported in *Gynecological Endocrinology*. Researchers found that women using 40 mg of transdermal progesterone cream a day for one year reported a significant reduction in hot flashes.

Other studies have shown that progesterone creams are also just as effective in increasing progesterone levels and easing menopausal symptoms as oral progestins—but significantly safer. According to a study presented at the annual meeting of the American Society for Clinical Pharmacology and Therapeutics, women given either natural progesterone cream or a synthetic oral progestin exhibited the same blood levels of the hormone.

A range of progesterone creams, available without a prescription, contain anywhere from less than 2 mg to more than 400 mg of the hormone per jar. Pro-Gest cream, which contains more than 400 mg in a container, is one of the better-known brands. The cream is applied to the skin and absorbed into the general circulation and reaches more body tissues than oral progesterone, which is first metabolized by the liver and converted into three different compounds.

A typical dosage of natural progesterone is 40 mg a day. A two-ounce jar should last for over one month. If you are perimenopausal, you should apply the cream from day 12 to day 26 of your menstrual cycle. If you are menopausal and not taking estrogen, you may use progesterone for two to three weeks each month, though some physicians do recommend daily use to avoid withdrawal bleeding.

If you are self-medicating with progesterone cream in an effort to block the cancer-promoting effect of estrogen on the uterus, you need to make sure you are taking enough progesterone for it to be protective. Blood or saliva testing of progesterone levels will help to determine if the level of supplemental progesterone you're using is in the therapeutic range.

The cream is used twice daily in 1/4-1/2 teaspoon amounts, generally upon rising in the morning and before going to bed at night. The cream can be applied to any area of the skin. Many women rub it into their chest, abdomen, arms, or back. If the cream is absorbed rapidly (under two minutes), it means that the body needs a higher dose, and a slightly higher amount may be used.

Note: Some reputed progesterone creams that contain wild yam extract contain only the precursor compound— diosgenin— and little to no progesterone. Also, progesterone delivered as a cream must suspend the hormone in a proper medium or it will not be effective. A cream containing mineral oil will not allow the progesterone to be absorbed properly. Some products have not stabilized the progesterone and, as a result, the hormone deteriorates over time.

Transdermal Sprays

Transdermal sprays work much like the creams, but without the mess. They are also quickly and efficiently absorbed into the skin with little need for rubbing. The spray also has a unique delivery system, which makes it easier to absorb than the cream.

A typical dosage of the spray is 5 to 10 sprays per day, usually upon rising in the morning and before going to bed at night. Like the cream, the spray can be applied to any area of the skin. I find that most women prefer to spray it on their arms, thighs, or abdomen. I am particularly partial to the ProgestEase brand of progesterone spray.

Sublingual Drops

Progesterone is available in a vitamin E oil base. This is held under the tongue for at least one minute so that it is absorbed, rather than swallowed. This results in a quick rise in hormone levels, followed by a drop three to four hours later. It is necessary to take the drops three to four times a day to maintain stable blood levels.

Suppositories

Progesterone can also be taken as a rectal or vaginal suppository. Vaginal suppositories allow for excellent local intake of progesterone into the uterus, and may be helpful for pre- or perimenopausal women with heavy and irregular bleeding.

Twenty five women with severe PMS and seventeen reproductive-age females participated in a controlled trial published in the *Journal of Assisted Reproduction and Genetics*. Treatment consisted of a 200 mg vaginal progesterone suppository, taken twice daily. The researchers observed that the women receiving the progesterone reported significant improvement in mood symptoms and nervousness.

A randomized, double-blind, placebo-controlled study published in *American Journal of Obstetrics and Gynecology* also found that the use of a vaginal progesterone suppository reduced the risk of preterm labor. Researchers gave 142 high-risk pregnant women either 100 mg of progesterone a day (administered by vaginal suppository) or a placebo. All were monitored for uterine contraction once a week for 60 minutes, between weeks 24 and 34 of gestation. They found that those women taking the progesterone had less uterine contractions that those receiving the placebo. They also found that less than 14 percent of the women in the progesterone group delivered early, and less than three percent delivered before 34 weeks, as compared to more than 18 percent of the placebo group delivering before 34 weeks.

Researchers concluded that progesterone suppositories reduce the frequency of uterine contractions and the threat of preterm delivery in high-risk women.

A number of studies have suggested that natural progesterone may be effective in protecting women from osteoporosis. John R. Lee, M.D., has done much research into the use of progesterone to reverse osteoporosis. The results of one of his studies were published in the *International Clinical Nutrition Review*.

As mentioned earlier in the book, Dr. Lee selected 100 Caucasian, postmenopausal women between the ages of 38 and 83. The average age was 65.2 at the beginning of the study. The majority of the women had already experienced some loss of height due to osteoporosis. They were instructed to use conjugated estrogen (0.3 to 0.625 mg per day for three weeks each month) and progesterone (a 3 percent topical cream applied daily to the skin for 12 days each month or during the last two weeks of estrogen use). The women were also given a dietary and exercise program to follow, as well as vitamin and mineral supplements. Alcohol consumption was limited, and no smoking was allowed. The bone health of the women was followed for at least three years.

All the women in the study experienced some degree of progressive increase in bone mineral density, as well as improvement in such clinical symptoms as height stabilization, pain relief, and an increase in physical activity. During the course of the study, there were also no fractures due to osteoporosis. These improvements occurred independent of the women's ages. The women commonly had an increase in the density of vertebral bone of 10 percent in the first six to 12 months of treatment. This increase was purportedly followed by additional yearly increases of 3 to 5 percent. This degree of bone remineralization over a relatively short period of time constitutes an exceptionally good therapeutic response.

Summary

Maintaining adequate progesterone levels benefits your mood, your sleep, and your overall health. By following the program I've described in the last two chapters, you can maintain this balance for years to come.

My program includes:

1. Stimulating progesterone production at the central nervous system level with 5-HTP, vitex, maca, and glandulars.
2. Promoting progesterone production in the ovaries with lutein, beta-carotene, flaxseed, and fish oil.
3. Using biochemically identical natural progesterone.

About Susan M. Lark, M.D.

Dr. Susan Lark is one of the foremost authorities in the fields of women's health care and alternative medicine. Dr. Lark has successfully treated many thousands of women emphasizing holistic health and complementary medicine in her clinical practice. Her mission is to provide women with unique, safe and effective alternative therapies to greatly enhance their health and well-being.

A graduate of Northwestern University Feinberg School of Medicine, she has served on the clinical faculty of Stanford University Medical School, and taught in their Division of Family and Community Medicine.

Dr. Lark is a distinguished clinician, author, lecturer and innovative product developer. She has been an innovator in the use of self-care treatments such as diet, nutrition, exercise and stress management techniques in the field of women's health. She is the author of many best-selling books on women's health. Her signature line of nutritional supplements and skin care products are available through healthydirections.com.

One of the most widely referenced physicians on the Internet, Dr. Lark has appeared on numerous radio and television shows, and has been featured in many magazines and newspapers.

She has also served as a consultant to major corporations, including the Kellogg Company and Weider Nutrition International, and was spokesperson for The Gillette Company Women's Cancer Connection.

Dr. Lark can be contacted at (650) 561-9978 to make an appointment for a consultation.

Dr. Susan's Solutions
Health Library For Women

The following books are available from iTunes, Amazon.com, Amazon Kindle, Womens Wellness Publishing and other major booksellers. Dr. Susan is frequently adding new books to her health library.

Women's Health Issues

Dr. Susan's Solutions: Healthy Heart and Blood Pressure

Dr. Susan's Solutions: Healthy Menopause

Dr. Susan's Solutions: The Anemia Cure

Dr. Susan's Solutions: The Bladder Infection Cure

Dr. Susan's Solutions: The Candida-Yeast Infection Cure

Dr. Susan's Solutions: The Chronic Fatigue Cure

Dr. Susan's Solutions: The Cold and Flu Cure

Dr. Susan's Solutions: The Endometriosis Cure

Dr. Susan's Solutions: The Fibroid Tumor Cure

Dr. Susan's Solutions: The Irregular Menstruation Cure

Dr. Susan's Solutions: The Menstrual Cramp Cure

Dr. Susan's Solutions: The PMS Cure

Emotional and Spiritual Balance

Breathing Meditations for Healing, Peace and Joy

Dr. Susan's Solutions: The Anxiety and Stress Cure

Women's Hormones

DHEA: The Fountain of Youth Hormone

Healthy, Natural Estrogens for Menopause

Pregnenolone: Your #1 Sex Hormone

Progesterone: The Superstar of Hormone Balance

Testosterone: The Hormone for Strong Bones, Sex Drive and Healthy Menopause

Diet and Nutrition

Dr. Susan Lark's Healing Herbs for Women

Dr. Susan Lark's Complete Guide to Detoxification

Enzymes: The Missing Link to Health

Healthy Diet and Nutrition for Women: The Complete Guide

Renew Yourself Through Juice Fasting and Detoxification Diets

Energy Therapies and Anti-Aging

Acupressure for Women: Relieve Symptoms of Dozens of Health Issues Through Pressure Points

Exercise and Flexibility

Stretching and Flexibility for Women

Stretching Programs for Women's Health Issues

About Womens Wellness Publishing

"Bringing Radiant Health and Wellness to Women"

Womens Wellness Publishing was founded to make a positive difference in the lives of women and their families. We are the premier publisher of print and eBooks focused on women's health and wellness. We are committed to publishing the finest quality and most comprehensive line of books that covers every area that a woman needs to create vibrant health and a joyful, fulfilling life.

Our books are written and created by the top health and wellness experts who share with you, our readers, their wisdom and extensive experience successfully treating many thousands of patients.

We encourage you to browse through our online bookstore; new books are frequently being added to womenswellnesspublishing.com. Visit our Lifestyle Center and Customer Bonus Center for more exciting and helpful health and wellness information and resources.

Follow us on Facebook for the latest health tips, recipes, and all natural solutions to many women's health issues (facebook.com/wwpublishing).

We would enjoy hearing from you! Please share your success stories, comments and requests for new topics at yourstory@wwpublishing.com.

About Our Associate Program

We invite you to become part of the Womens Wellness Publishing Community through our Associate Program. You will have the opportunity to earn generous commissions on sales that you create through your blog, social network, support groups, community groups, school & alumni groups, friends, family or other networks.

To join the Associate Program, go to our website, womenswellnesspublishing.com, and click "Become an Associate"

We support your sales and marketing efforts by offering you and your customers:

- Free support materials with updates on all of our new book releases, promotions, and bonuses for you and your customers
- Free audio downloads, booklets, and guides
- Special discounts and sales promotions

Made in the USA
Lexington, KY
09 June 2013